ISBN-13: 978-1508992196

ISBN-10: 1508992193

A special thanks to my wife for her encouragement and support and to the countless children who I have spoken to over the years at various elementary schools who helped to inspire me even more to write a book that would motivate children to exercise in a fun way.

To my first born son, Mason, who as a child spent hours in my personal training studio watching me and then when he was old enough, tried to pick up his first weight to mimic what I was doing. I could see early on the importance of parents setting good examples in the areas of   exercise and healthy eating. When people say, "Like father like son", they are more right then wrong. Even more so when we bring a child up into an environment that promotes physical activities.

Ron Henderson can be contacted at: Email: baldking@gmail.com

Phone: 612-386-8178

Address: Ron Henderson

4301 Highway 7 Suite 110

St. Louis Park, MN 55416

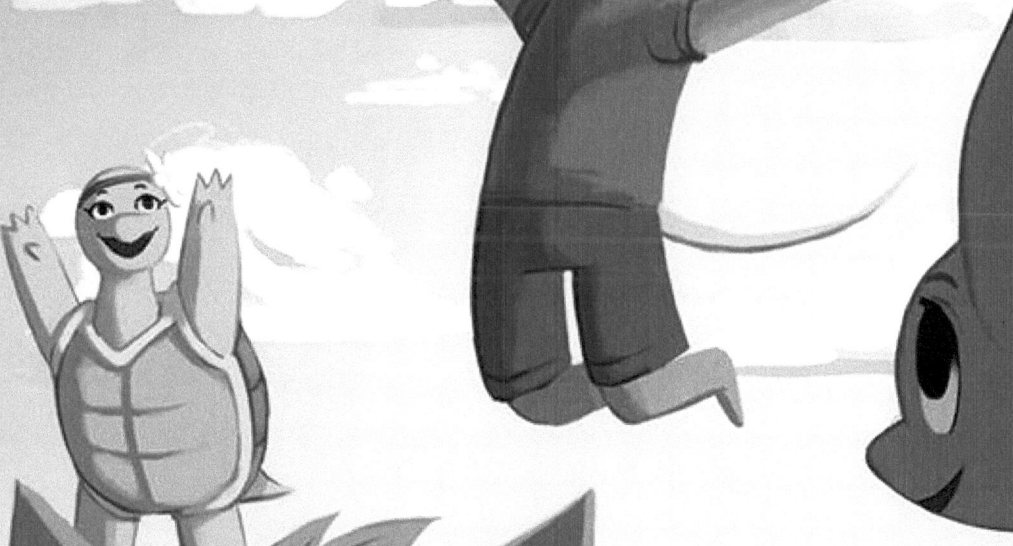

MASON'S BACKYARD WORKOUT!

BY RON HENDERSON "THE FITNESS KING"

Illustrated by LIZZY STAMPHER

MASON'S BACKYARD WORKOUT by Ron Henderson "The Fitness King"

This book originated over 22 years ago with a dream to publish a children's book about a Mouse that decides to have a backyard workout get-together with all of his animal friends. Now this dream is a reality with this first book of the Mason the Mouse series.

Over the past 35 years I have been to numerous elementary schools and the one thing that seemed to be common among the children was that they liked to exercise and even more when it was fun. Now, with the increase in iPhones, iPads, the internet and so on, kids have become less active.

When my first child was born, I realized that he was more active than most kids his age—mostly because he grew up in my personal training gym and in a household that believed in the importance of taking care of one's health. With that in mind, and countless visits to area elementary schools, I was determined to write a book that would teach children the
importance of moving and stretching. I am declaring to leave no child behind and crack the code on childhood obesity. When you read this book to your children they will hear about exercise in a fun way.

.

After spending the day cleaning his room,
Mason washed his hands and put away his broom.
Now that his chores were done, Mason could rest
or do something fun!

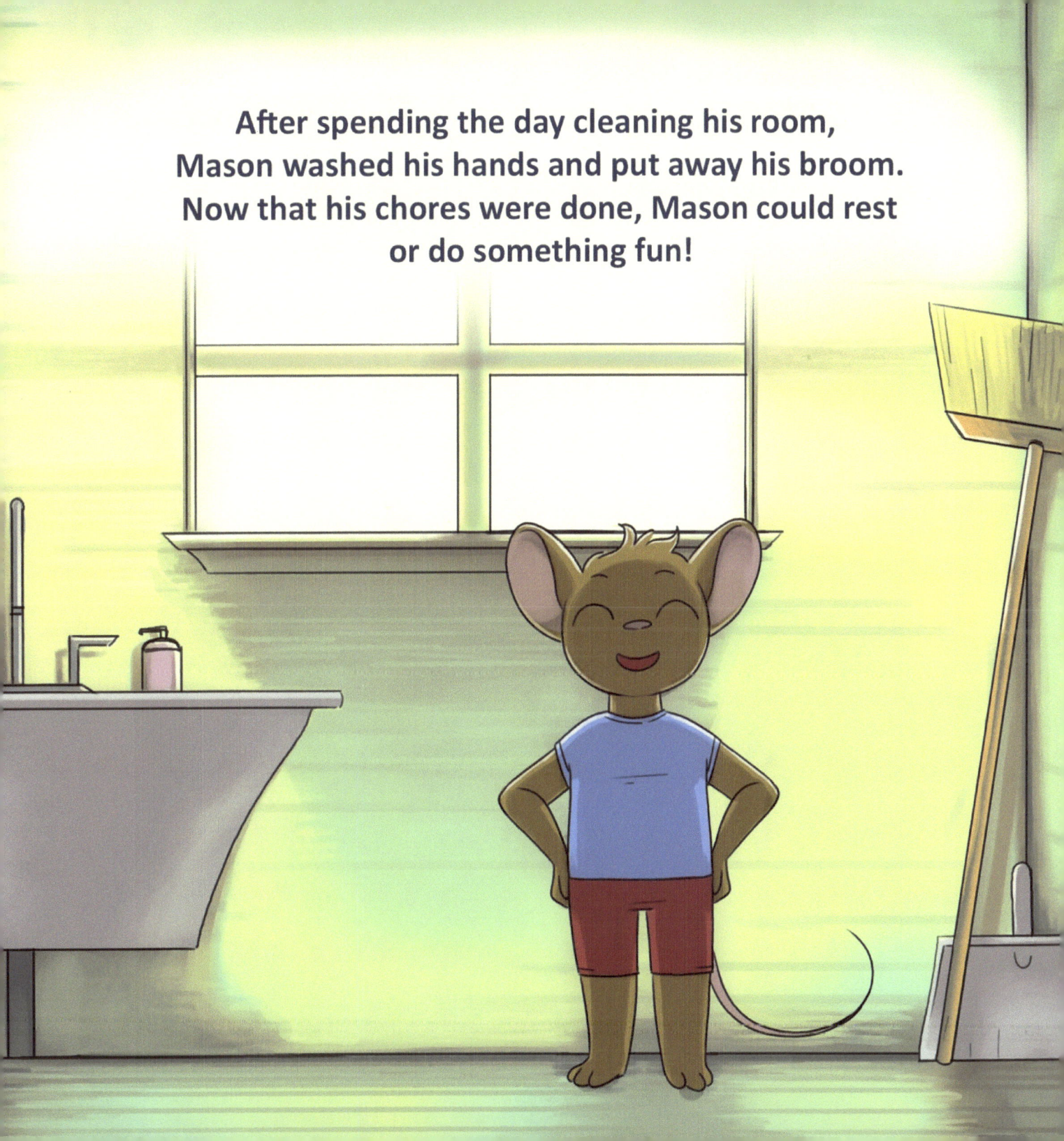

With the TV turned on he decided to sit.
He'd watch a show or read a bit.
As he sat on the couch a commercial came on
talking about making our bodies healthy and strong!

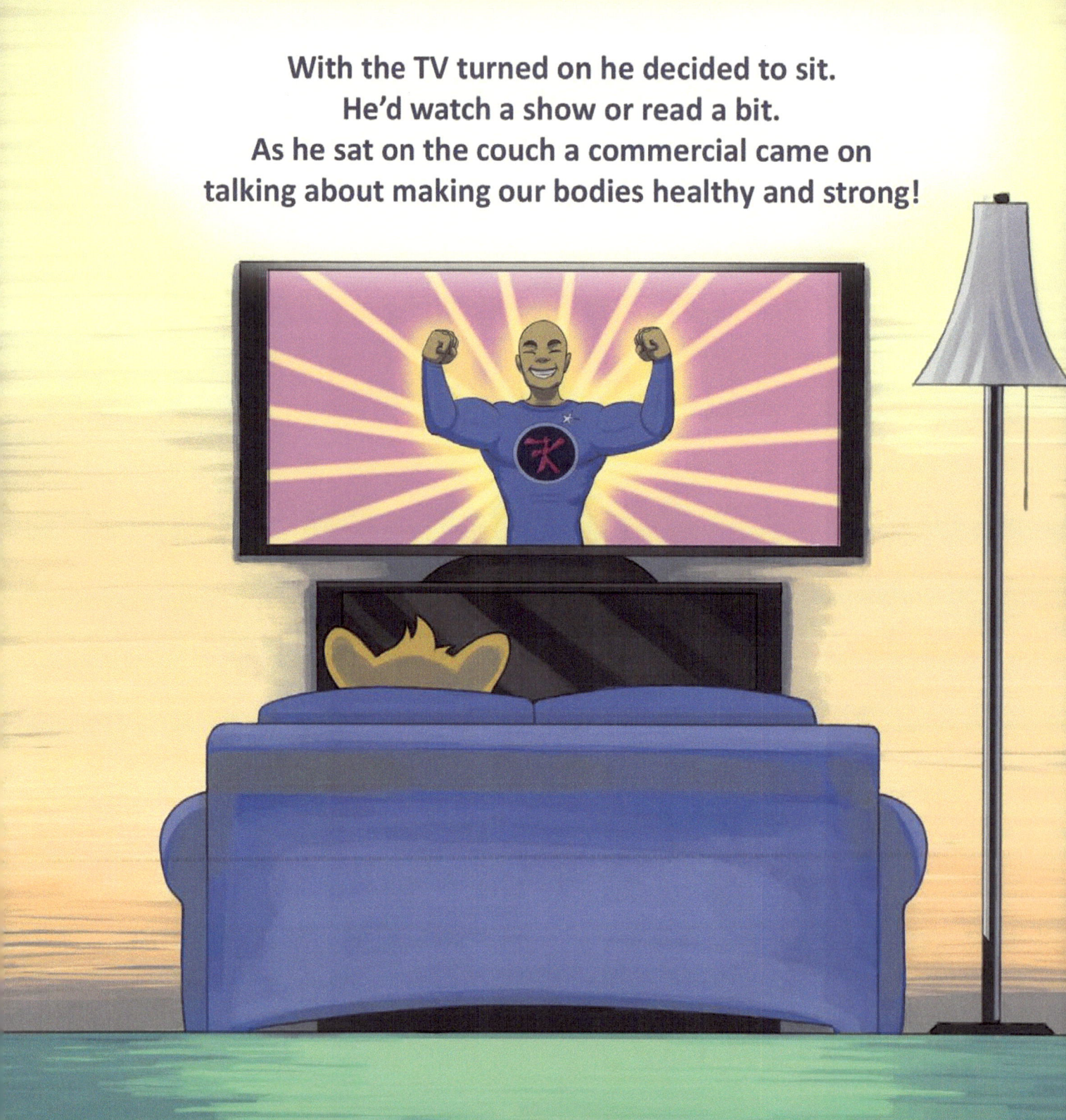

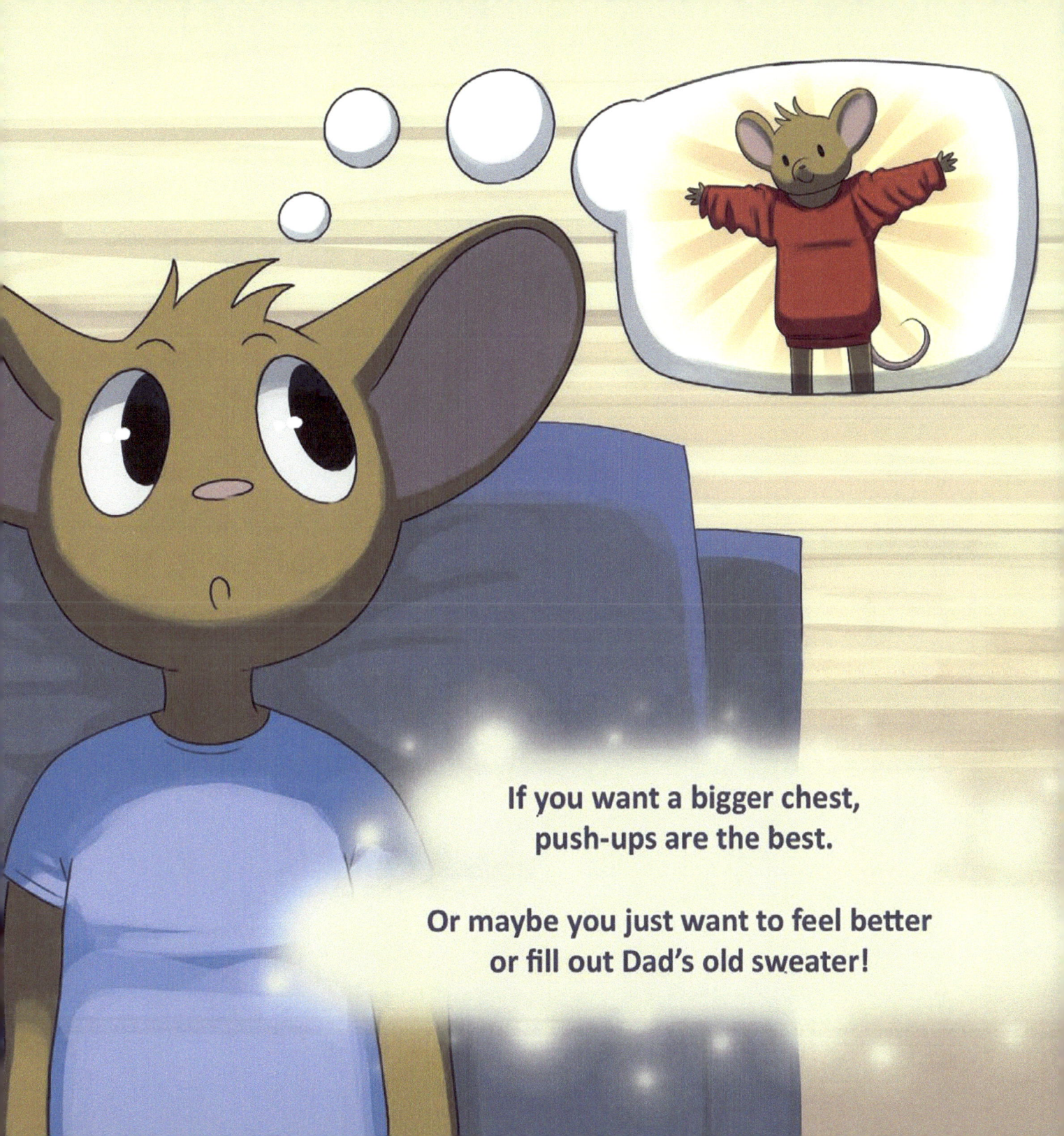

As Mason listened to the man on TV talking,
he got off the couch and started walking.
Forward and back, with his eyes on the screen,
he imagined his friends all looking lean.

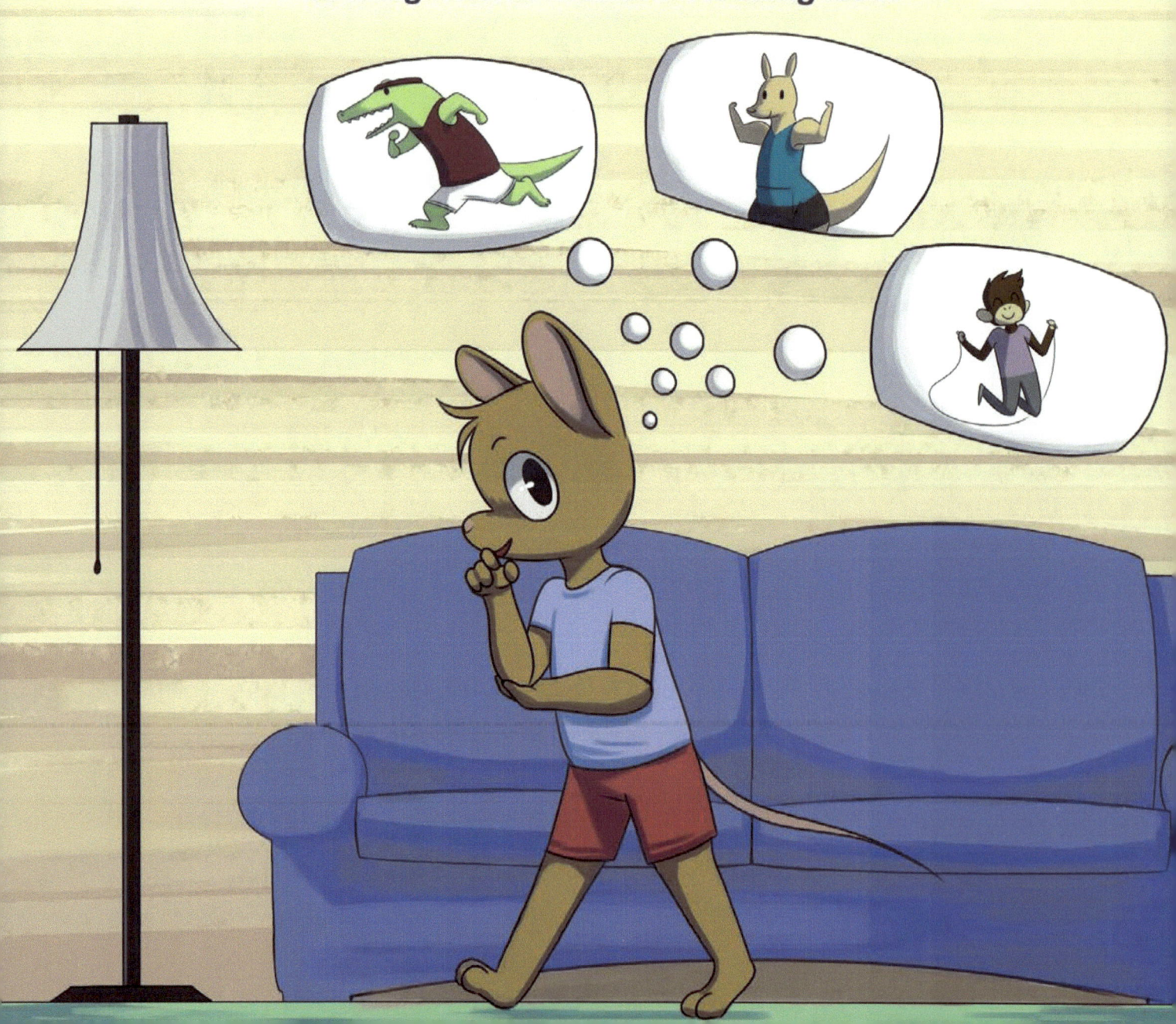

If they were stronger, he thought,
they could play longer!

If they had more energy they could go for long walks,
not just down the driveway but all around the
block.

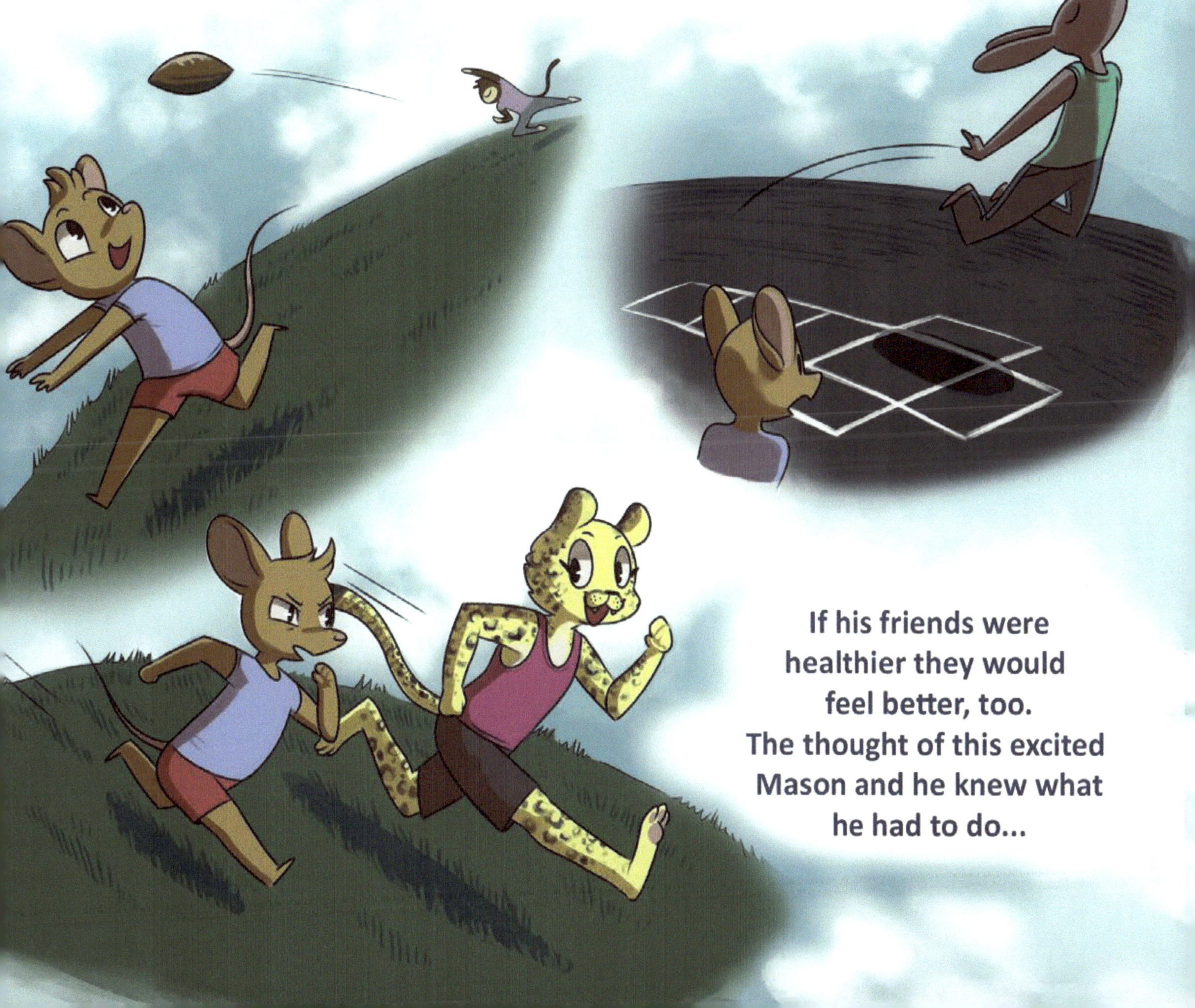

If his friends were
healthier they would
feel better, too.
The thought of this excited
Mason and he knew what
he had to do...

A back yard workout he would plan, and invite all the animals in the land!
His friend, Ellen the eagle, will help get the word out.
She will drop off cards that say,
"Come to Mason's Backyard Workout!"

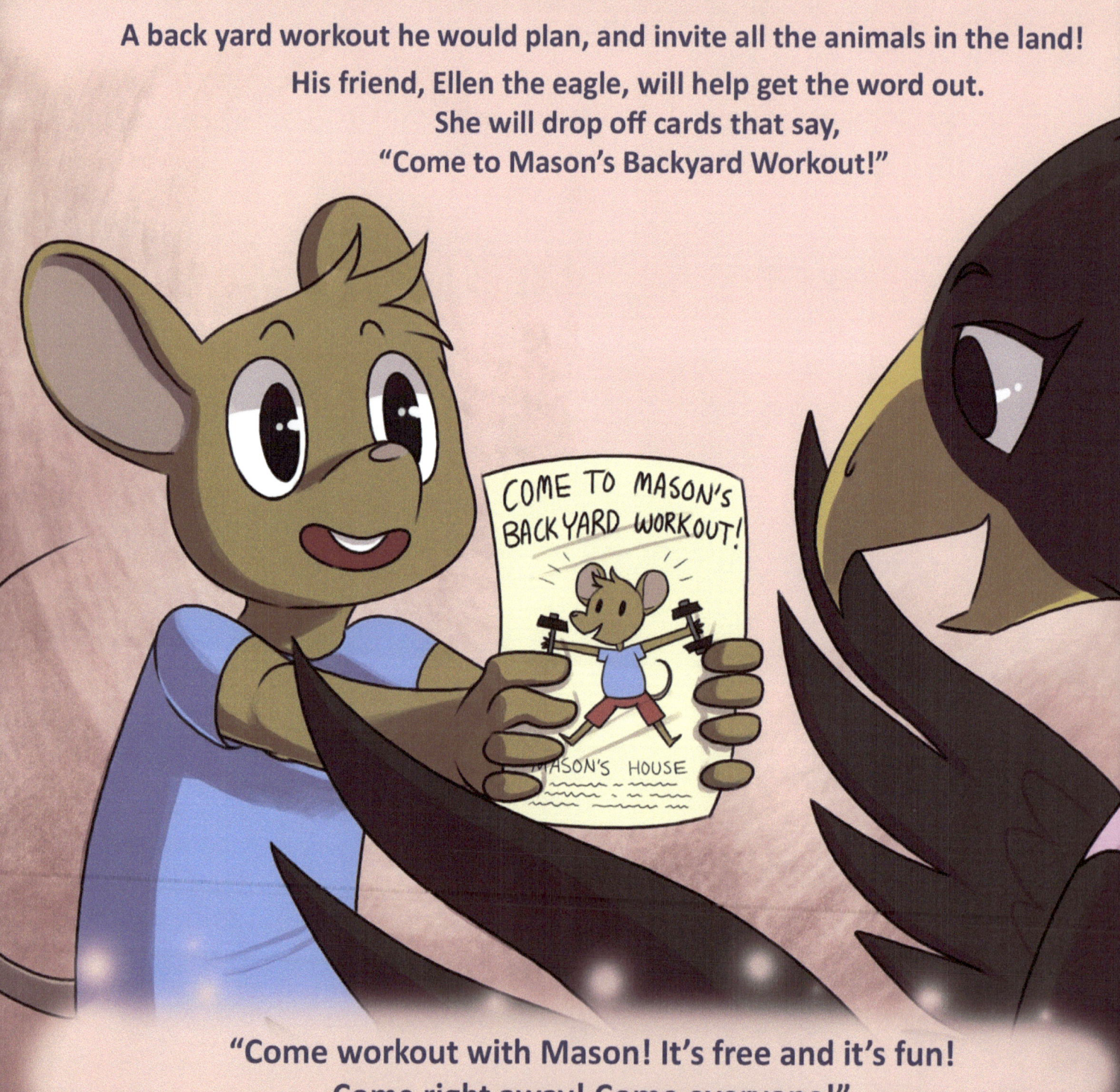

"Come workout with Mason! It's free and it's fun!
Come right away! Come everyone!"

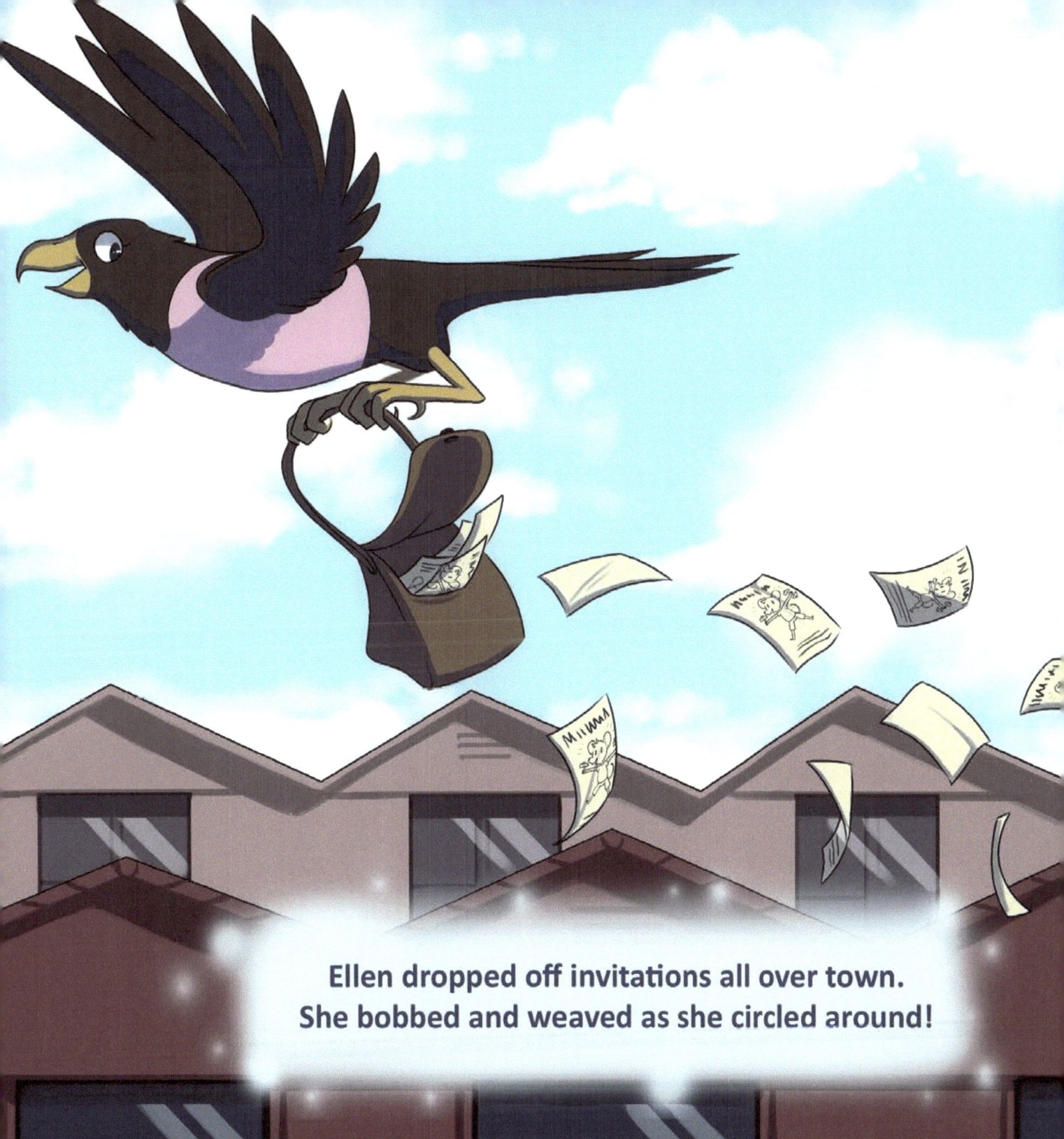

Ellen dropped off invitations all over town.
She bobbed and weaved as she circled around!

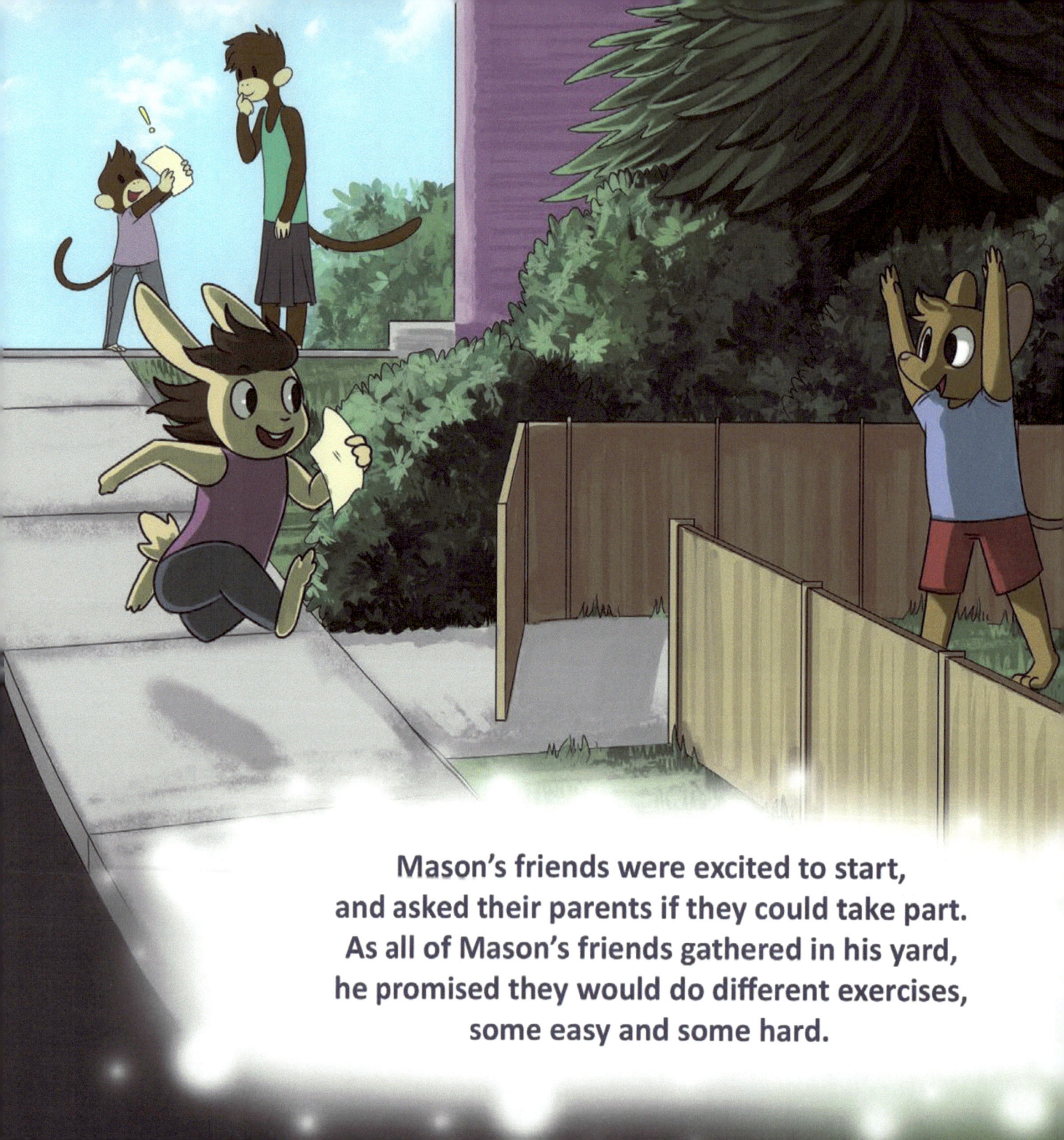

Mason's friends were excited to start,
and asked their parents if they could take part.
As all of Mason's friends gathered in his yard,
he promised they would do different exercises,
some easy and some hard.

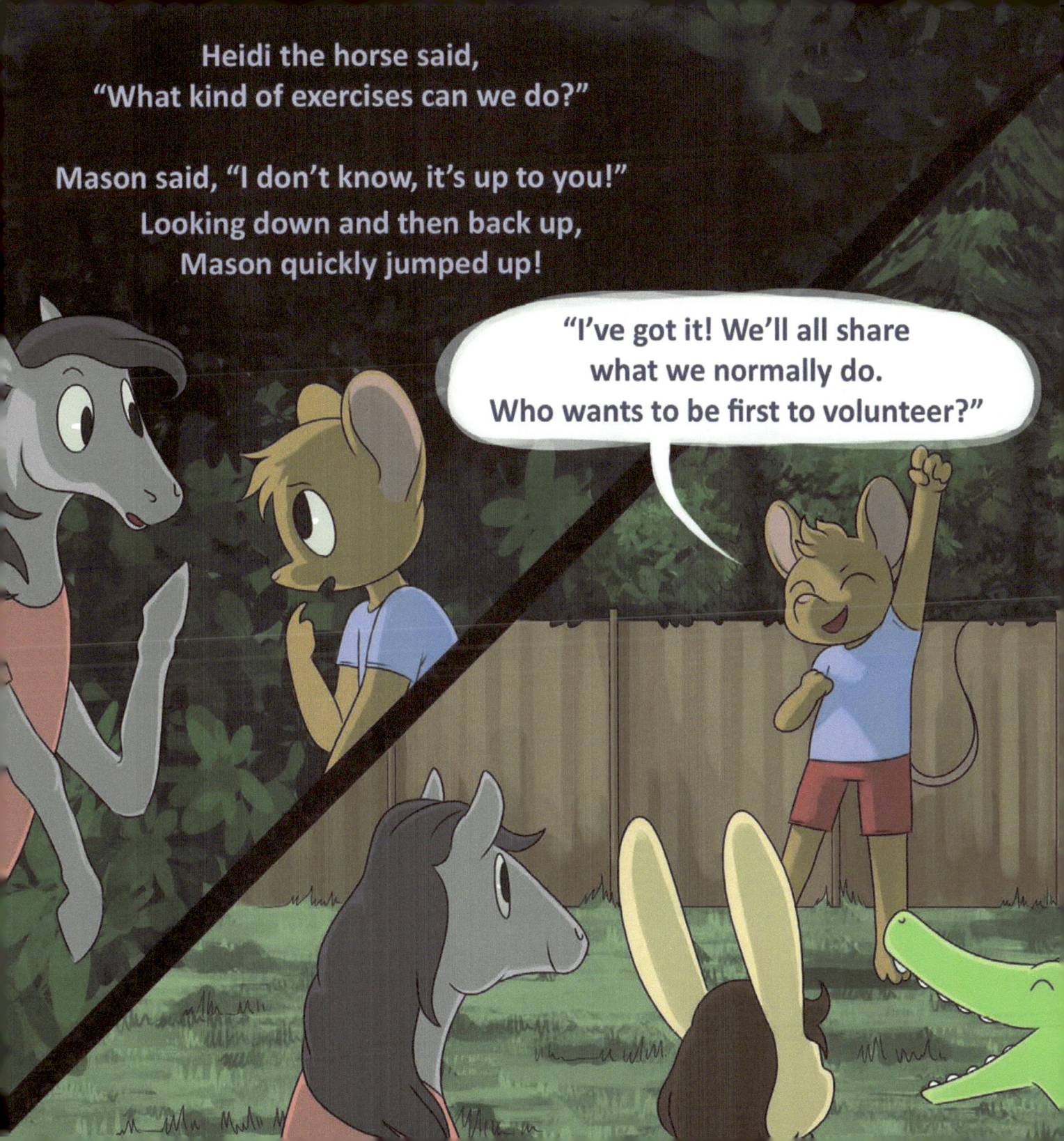

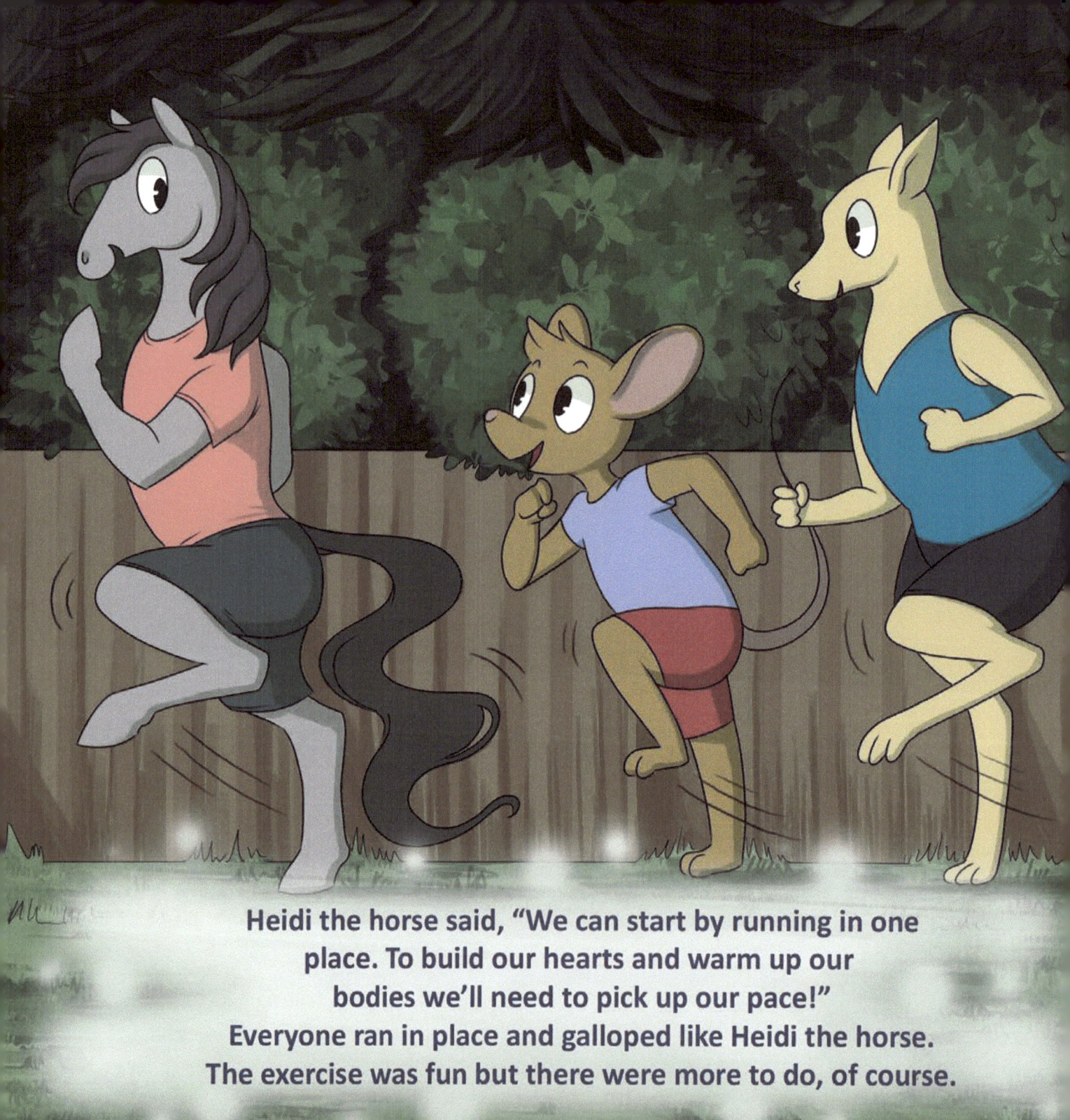

Heidi the horse said, "We can start by running in one place. To build our hearts and warm up our bodies we'll need to pick up our pace!"
Everyone ran in place and galloped like Heidi the horse.
The exercise was fun but there were more to do, of course.

As he looked at the crowd he could see
Heidi the horse, Kay the kangaroo, Ellen the eagle,
Lionel the lioness, Petey the puppy dog, Bailey the cat,
Mona the butterfly and many more...
All waiting to do the next exercise.

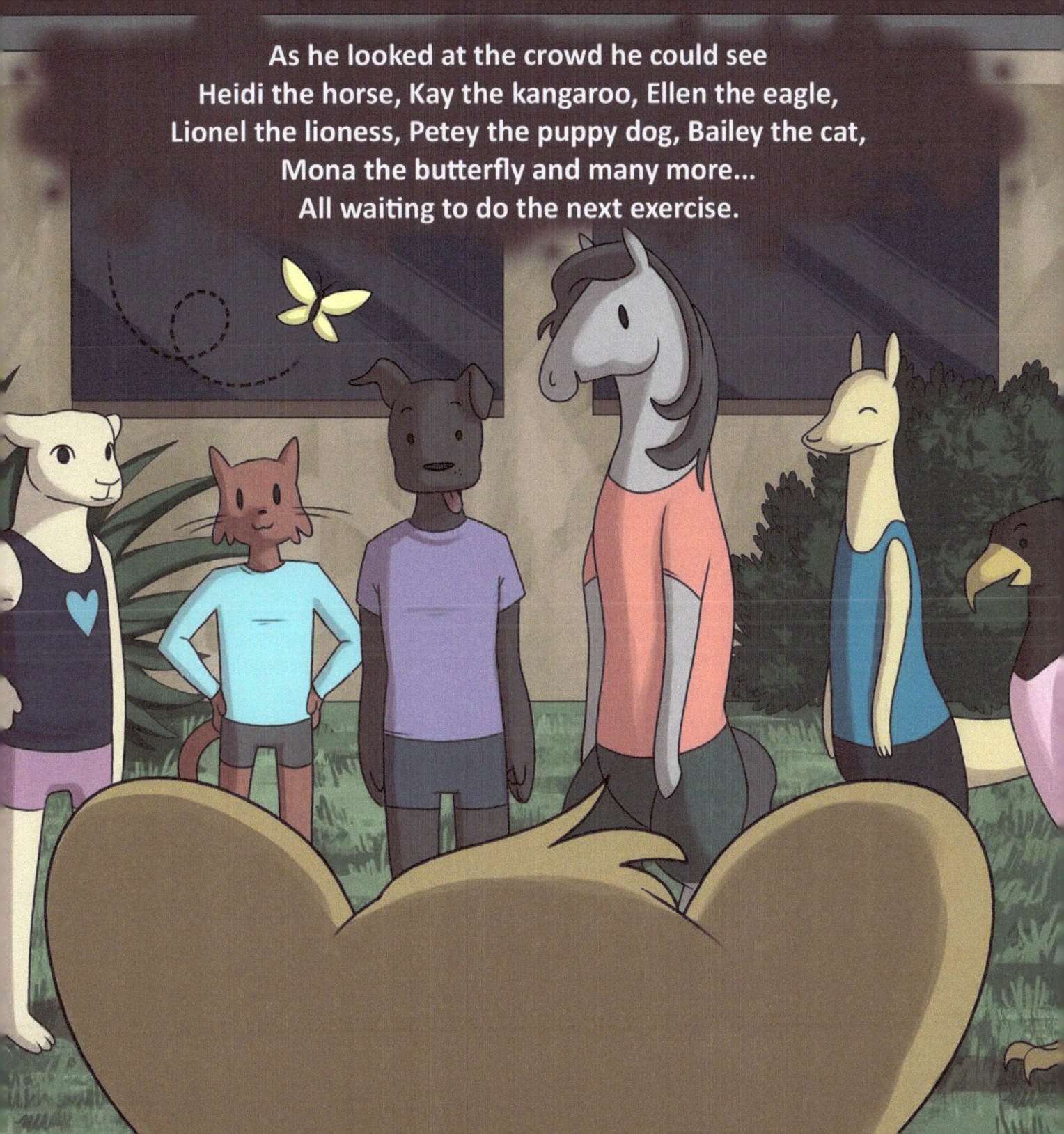

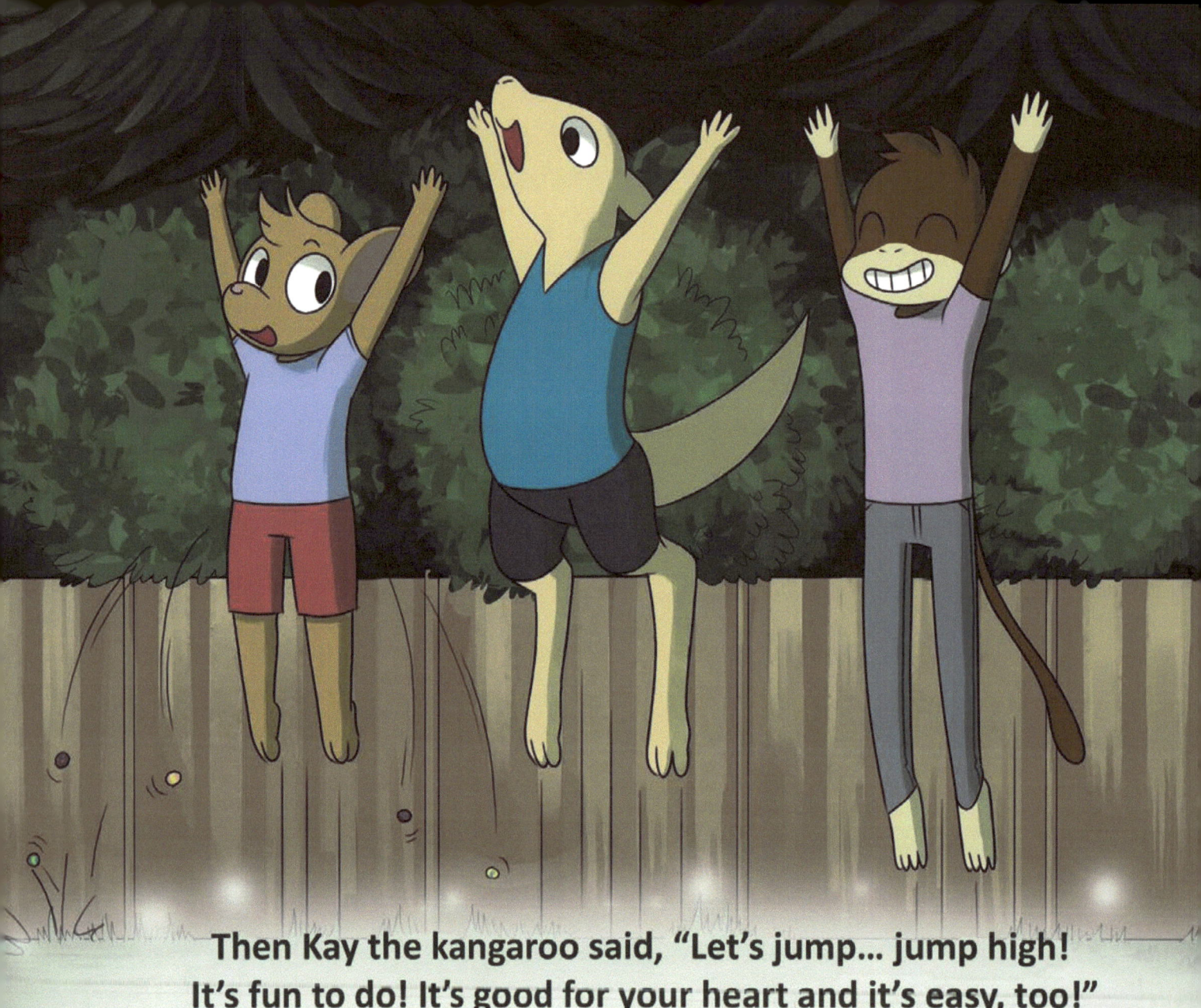

Then Kay the kangaroo said, "Let's jump... jump high!
It's fun to do! It's good for your heart and it's easy, too!"
Mason was jumping so fast that his marbles fell out of his pockets!

Everyone jumped in place for 30 seconds and not a second shorter,
or a second more, for no one knew what was in store.
Although a little out of breath, everyone tried to do their best!

Marty the monkey yelled to Mason, "I've got one, watch me!"
He jumped up on the closest branch and hung from the
big green tree. Everybody grabbed a tree branch and
let their bodies hang to stretch out their muscles
and feel long and lean.

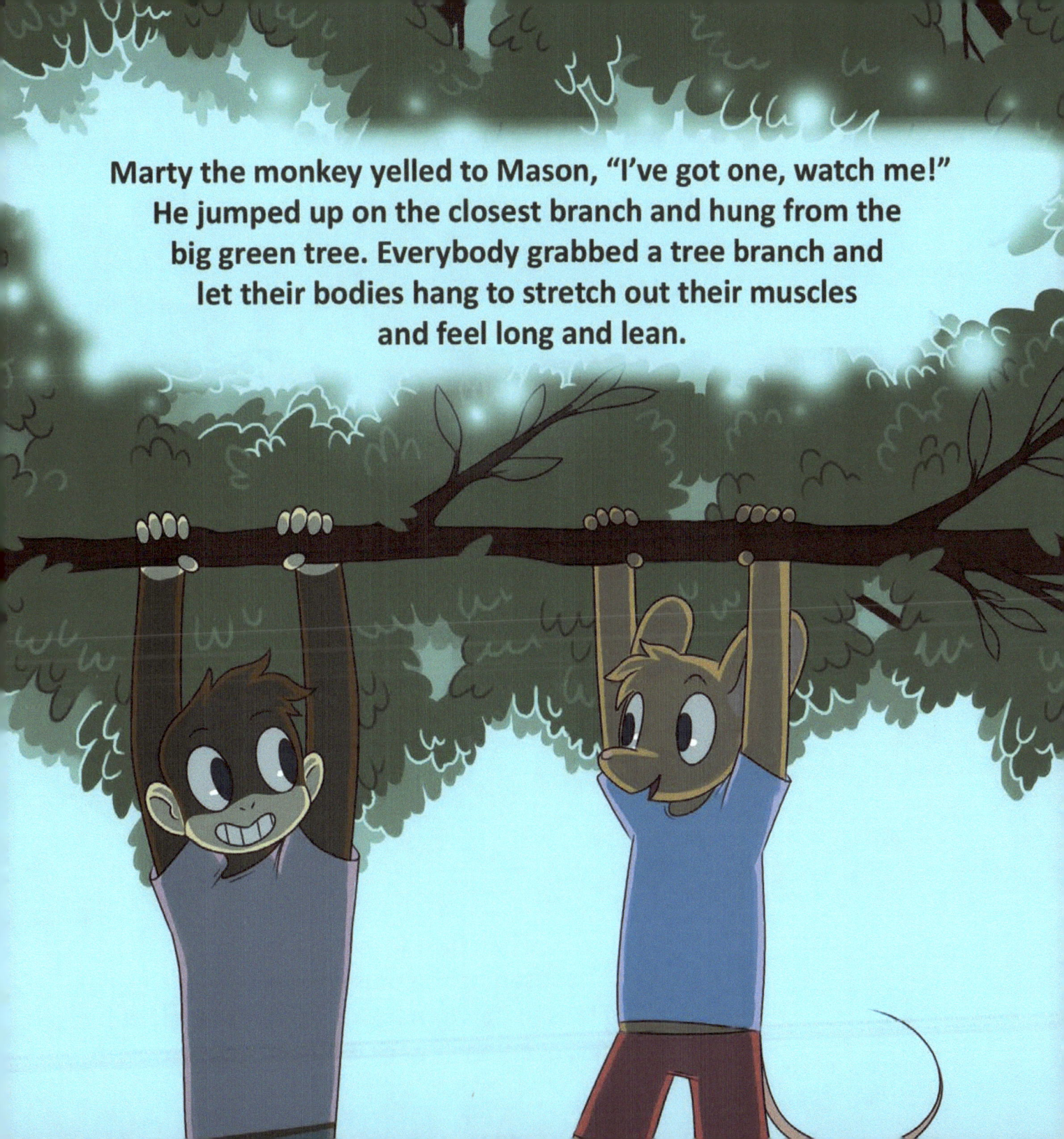

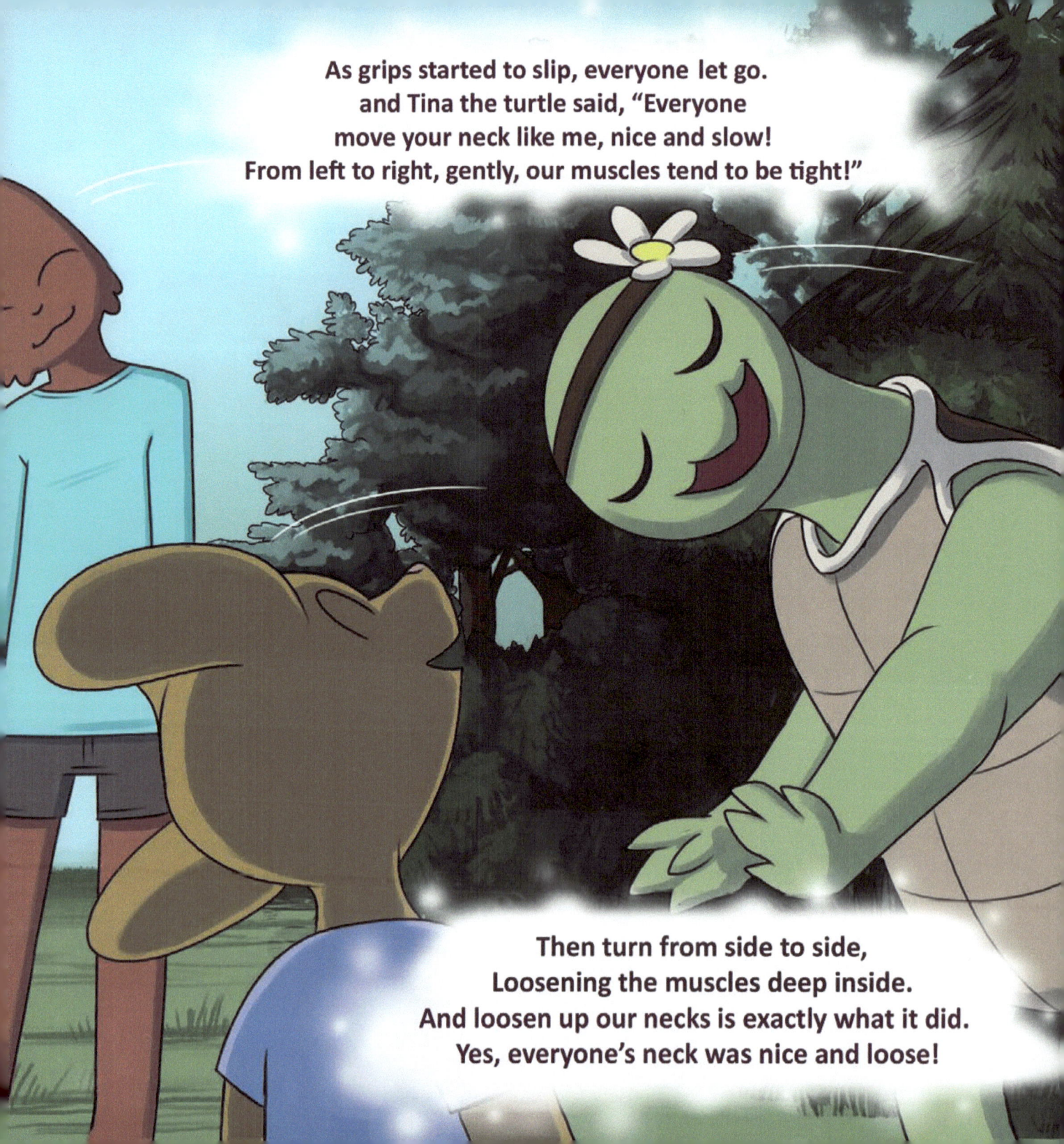

As grips started to slip, everyone let go.
and Tina the turtle said, "Everyone
move your neck like me, nice and slow!
From left to right, gently, our muscles tend to be tight!"

Then turn from side to side,
Loosening the muscles deep inside.
And loosen up our necks is exactly what it did.
Yes, everyone's neck was nice and loose!

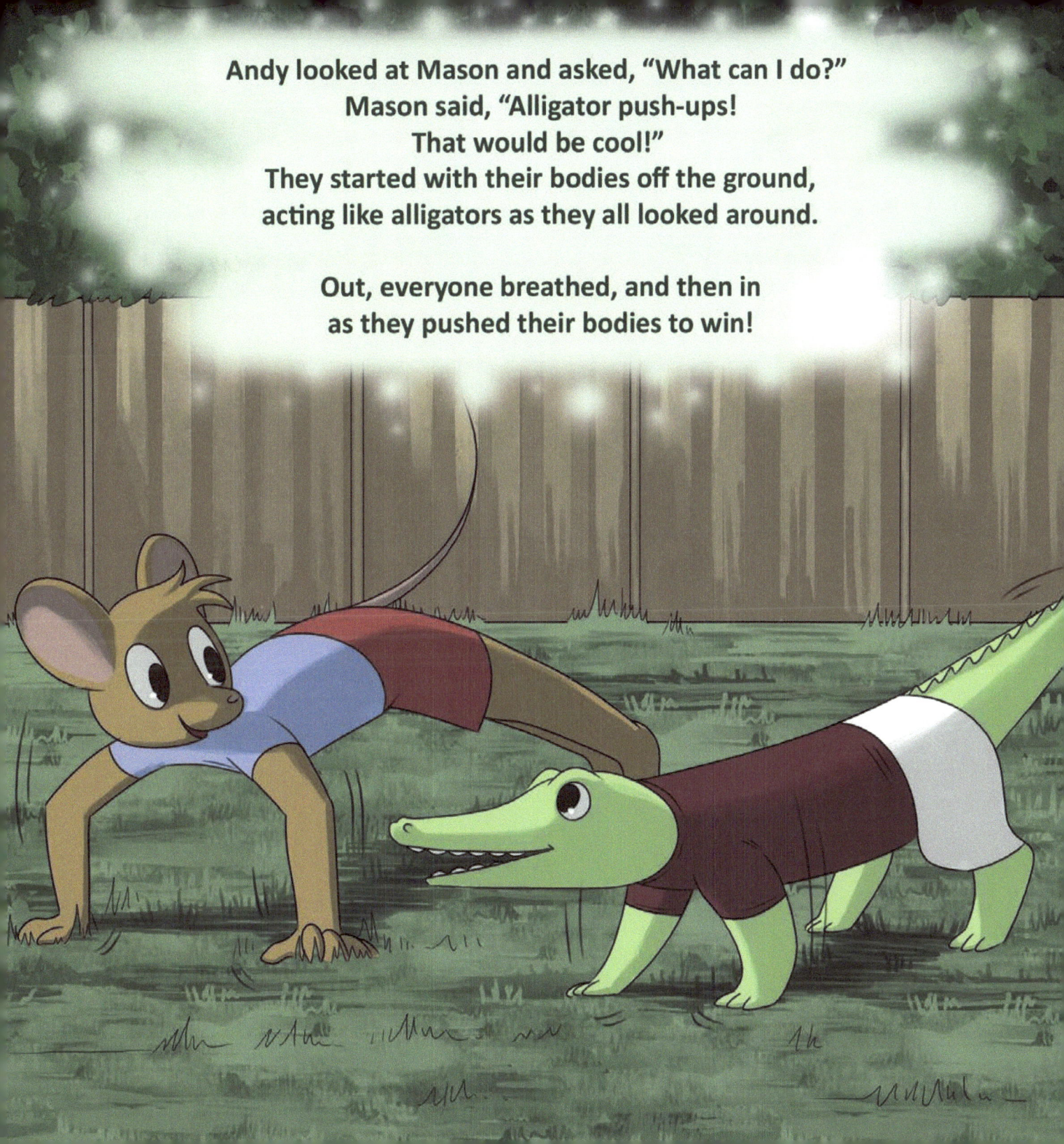

Andy looked at Mason and asked, "What can I do?"
Mason said, "Alligator push-ups!
That would be cool!"
They started with their bodies off the ground,
acting like alligators as they all looked around.

Out, everyone breathed, and then in
as they pushed their bodies to win!

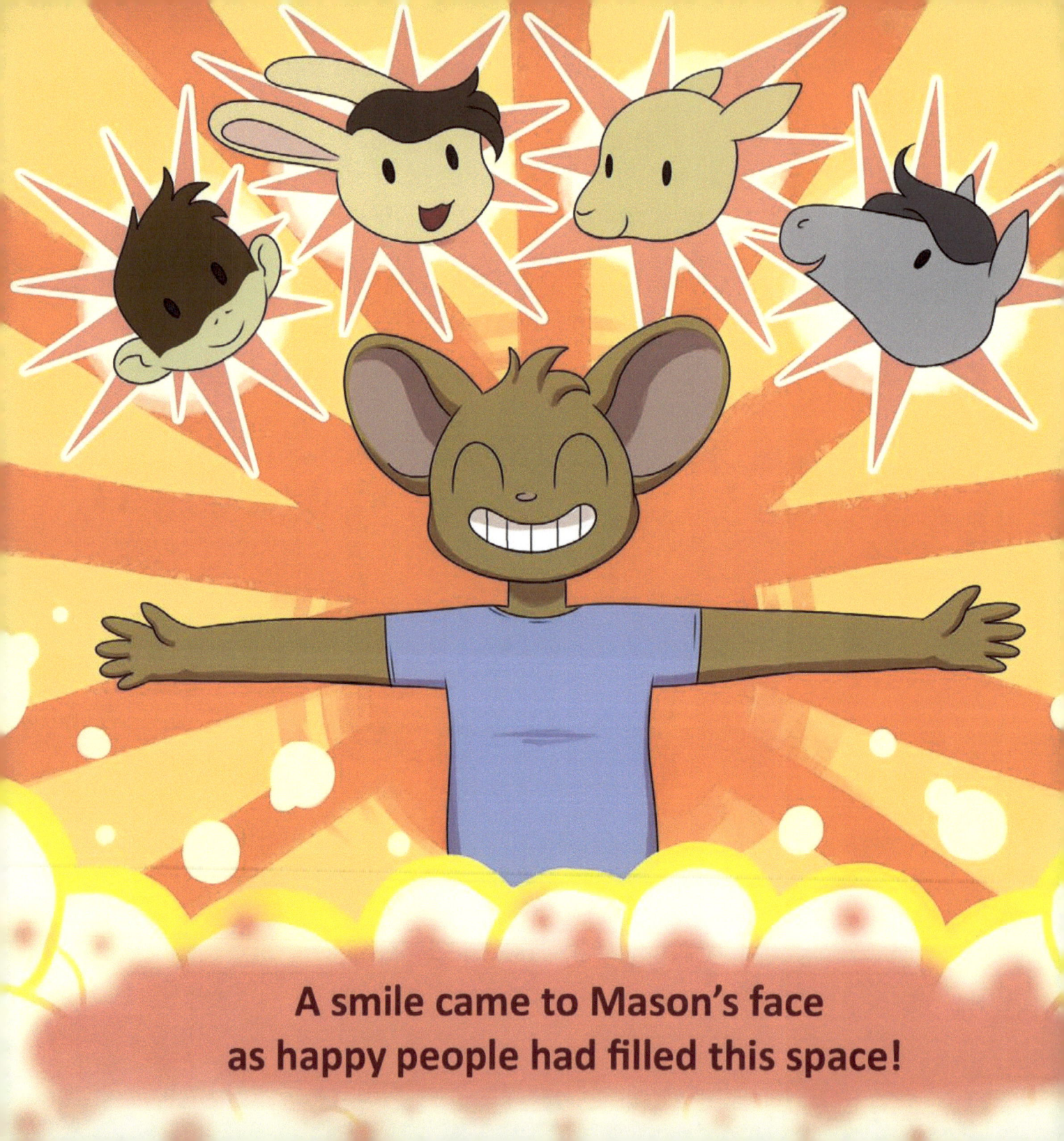

A smile came to Mason's face
as happy people had filled this space!

Everyone was having fun,
as Ellie tried to get her
push-ups done.

With her big trunk
in the way,
she pushed up and down
as her long trunk
swayed.

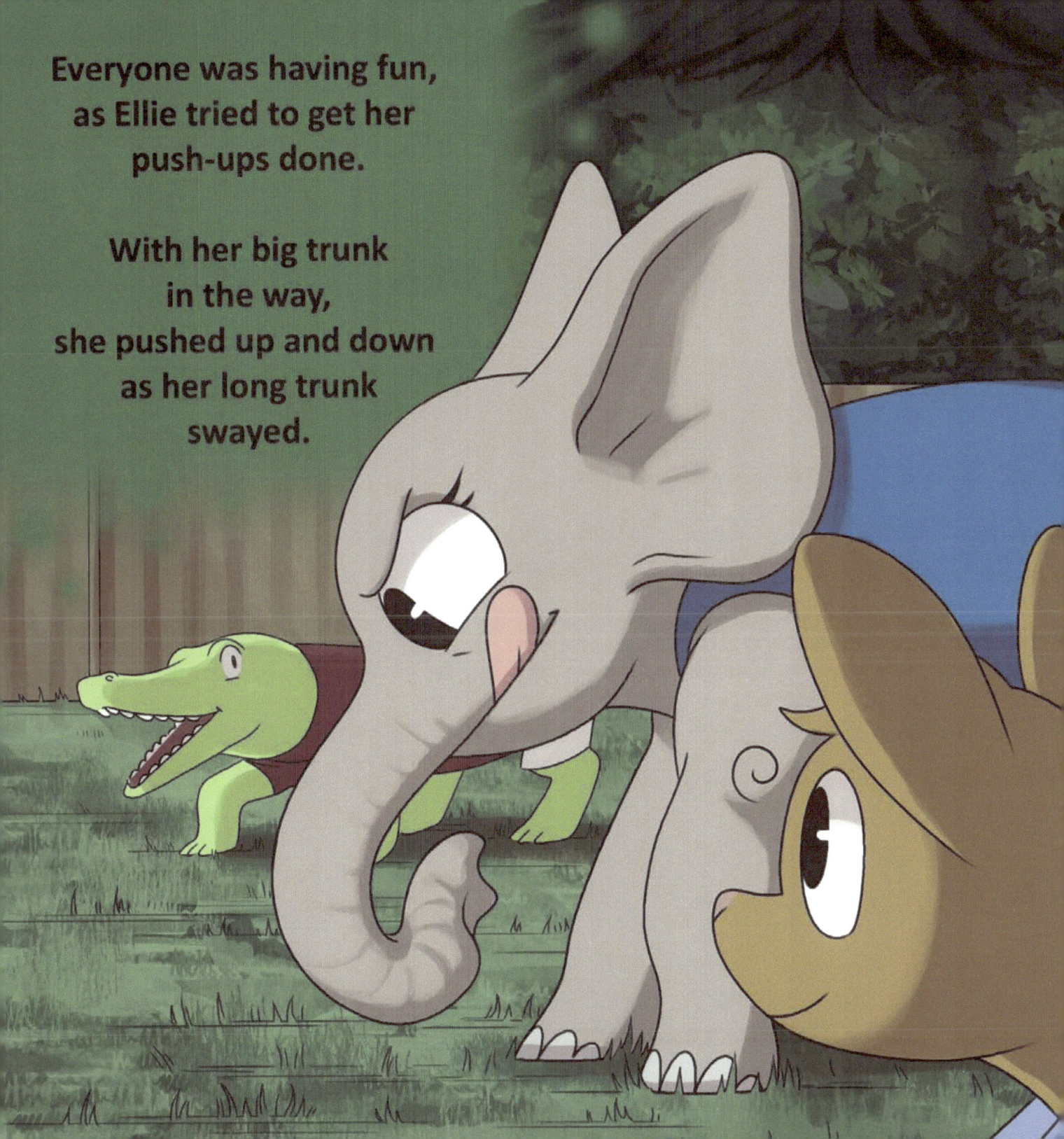

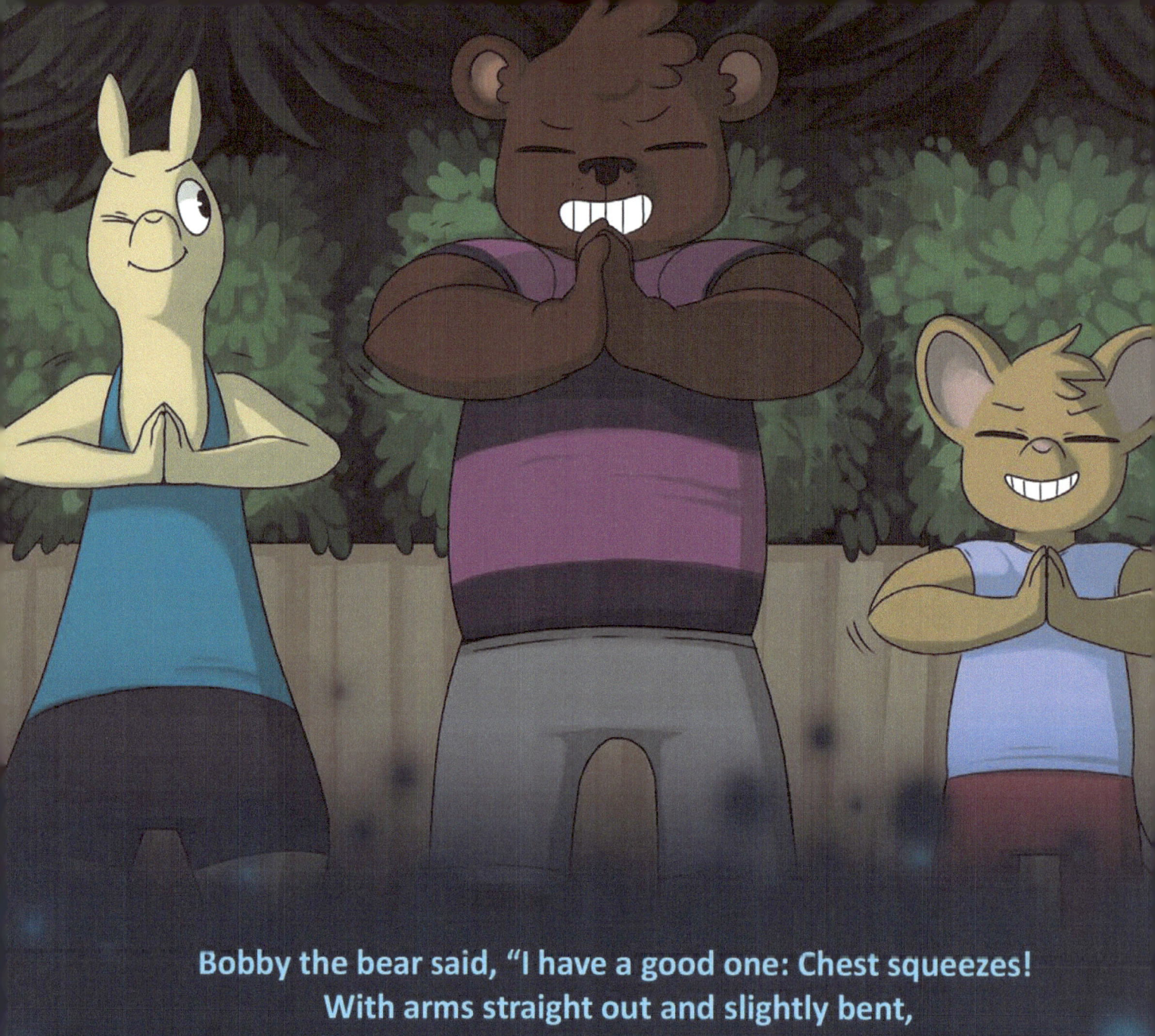

Bobby the bear said, "I have a good one: Chest squeezes!
With arms straight out and slightly bent,
like you're wrapping them around a tree.
Now cross them in front and squeeze for a few seconds
and relax, and squeeze again, and relax.
Repeat 5 times and you're set!"

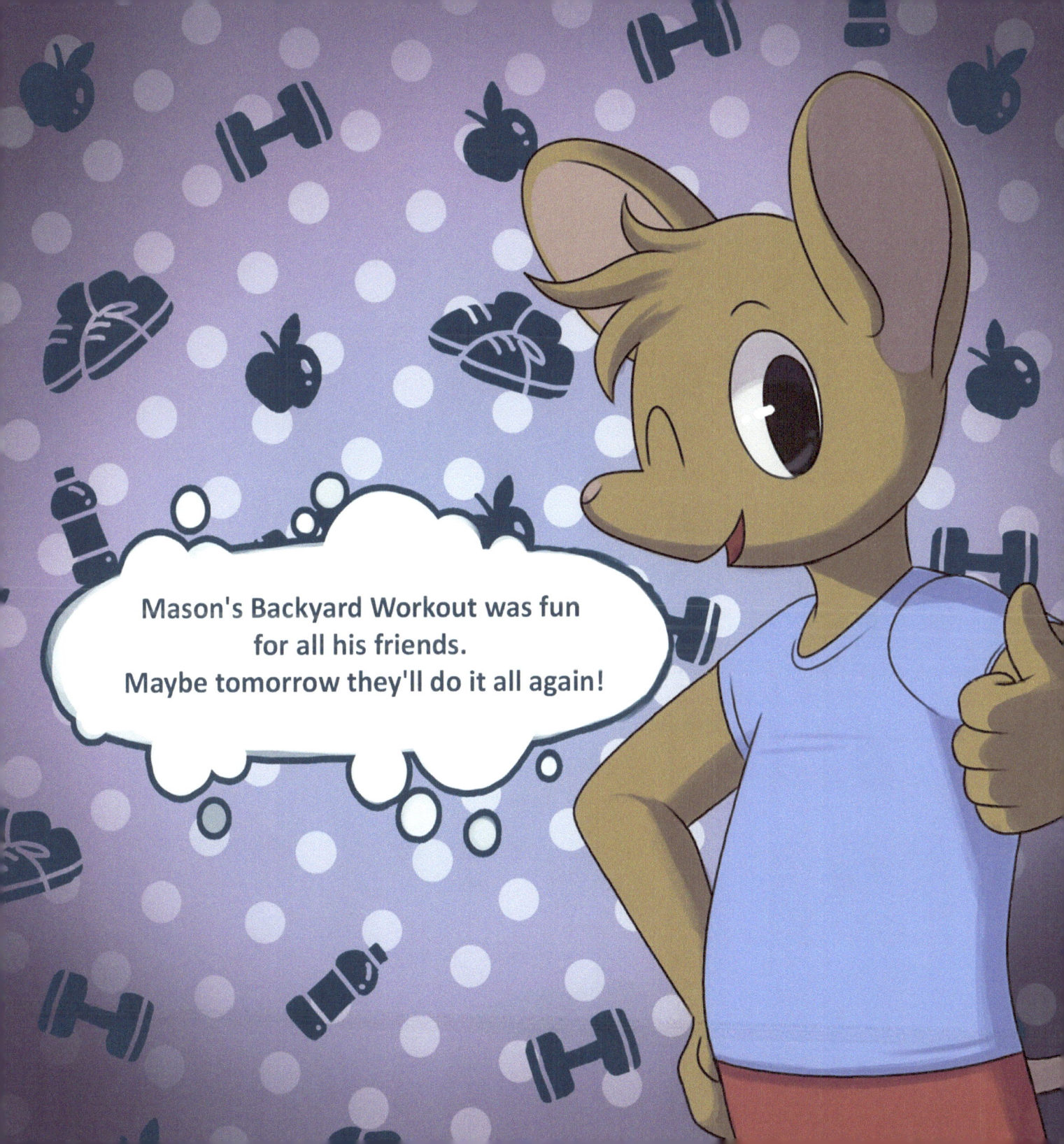

Who is Ron Henderson?

Ron Henderson, AKA the Fitness King, is a renowned personal trainer, motivational speaker and writer who has been the premier personal fitness trainer in the Twin Cities for over 35 years. His expertise has landed him interviews with numerous newspapers, magazines, radio stations and TV programs. Ron is the author of *What is it Worth for You to Become Physically Fit?*, *Fitness Economics*, and Fitness and Faith*: Balancing the Scales*. He has hosted the cable TV show *The King and the Kids* which was geared to motivate all children to get up and move.

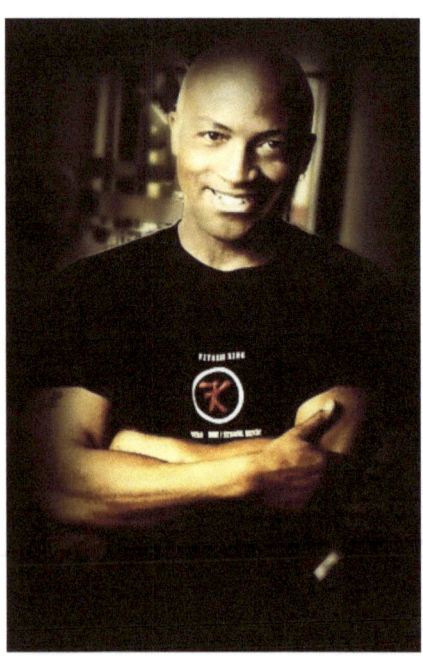

Draw your own exercises on these pages and invite your friends over for your very own backyard workout.